COGNITIVE

BEHAVIORAL

THERAPY

21 Great Ways to Deal with Anxiety, Depression, Worry and Panic

including specific information will be considered an illegal act irrespective of if it is done electronically or in print. This extends to creating a secondary or tertiary copy of the work or a recorded copy and is only allowed with an express written consent from the Publisher. All additional rights reserved.

The information in the following pages is broadly considered a truthful and accurate account of facts. As such, any inattention, use, or misuse of the information in question by the reader will render any resulting actions solely under their purview. There are no scenarios in which the publisher or the original author of this work can be in any fashion deemed liable for any hardship or damages that may befall them after undertaking information described herein.

Additionally, the information in the following pages is intended only for informational purposes and should thus be thought of as universal. As befitting its nature, it is presented without assurance regarding its prolonged validity or interim quality. Trademarks that are mentioned are done without written consent and can in no way be considered an endorsement from the trademark holder.

Table of Contents

INTRODUCTION

This book contains information on Cognitive Behavioral Therapy as well as pointers on how to effectively deal with anxiety, depression, worry, panic, and fears using various strategies. It contains details on how CBT works and its effects on your thoughts, feelings, and behaviors.

Here, you will learn about 21 practical ways on how to improve your condition and handle your situation better. These techniques contain step by step instructions as well as information on how they work. They are also backed up by scientific studies and research, which proves that they are safe and effective.

In addition, this book contains tips on how to prevent and overcome smoking, addictions, and phobias. It also tells you how you can change your core beliefs so that you can replace negative and limiting thoughts with positive and helpful ones. It also provides information on goal setting and mindfulness, which can further help you improve yourself, attain your goals, and live the kind of life that you want.

Keep in mind that it is never too late to make a change. You can always turn things around and get what you deserve. You are worthy of good health, happiness, and success.

Thanks for downloading this book, I hope you enjoy it!

CHAPTER 1

WHAT IS COGNITIVE BEHAVIORAL THERAPY?

Cognitive behavioral therapy is a kind of psychotherapy that modifies dysfunctional thoughts, emotions, and behaviors to treat issues and improve wellbeing. It focuses on finding solutions to encourage patients to change their destructive behavioral patterns as well as challenge their distorted cognitions. It is different from the traditional Freudian psychoanalysis approach, which digs deep into childhood to uncover past wounds that may be connected to the present problem.

It can be said that cognitive behavioral therapy is a combination of psychotherapy, which puts emphasis on the importance of personal meanings and childhood patterns; and behavioral therapy, which focuses on the relationship between thoughts, behaviors, and problems. Psychotherapists usually tailor the therapy to suit the specific needs and personalities of their patients.

Cognitive behavioral therapy is based on the theory that perceptions and thoughts affect behaviors. In certain situations, feelings of distress distort perception of reality. With cognitive behavioral therapy, harmful thoughts can be identified and evaluated. If they are found to be inaccurate depictions of reality, they can be modified through effective strategies.

Who Can Benefit from Cognitive Behavioral Therapy?

Anyone can benefit from cognitive behavioral therapy, regardless of age or gender. It is appropriate for adults, children, and adolescents with major depressive disorder, eating disorders, anxiety disorders, and other conditions. It is also helpful for individuals who are dealing with relationship problems, sleeping difficulties, addiction, and emotional problems.

How Can Treatment Be Obtained?

Traditionally, treatment is given in person. The patient has to see the therapist face-to-face. There are individual sessions, wherein the patient has a one-on-one conversation with the therapist, and group sessions, wherein the patient works with a group of individuals who have similar issues.

Today, however, modern techniques are also applied. For instance, using the Internet has been found to be convenient and effective. Patients can opt for online therapy in which they can talk to the therapist via e-mail, chat, or video call.

Cognitive behavioral therapy tends to be brief, only done for five to ten months. Patients can attend weekly sessions, with one session lasting for about fifty minutes. The therapists and patients should work hand in hand to understand the problems and find solutions. They should also develop strategies that can help them effectively deal with the problem for life.

You can go to the National Association of Cognitive Behavioral Therapists to check out the directory of certified cognitive behavioral therapists. You can also use Psych Central's Therapist Finder.

Thoughts, Beliefs, and Cognitive Behavioral Therapy

Cognitive behavioral therapy is based on the theory that events do not upset people, but rather the meanings they attach to such events. So, if your thoughts are negative, they can prevent you from having a wider perspective and doing things differently. You become stuck and hold on to the same limiting beliefs.

For example, if you are depressed, you may think that you cannot come in to work today because you are not good enough. You may think that your day will turn out to be awful. Because of such negative thoughts, you do not come in to work and you miss out on the chance to see if your predictions are wrong. By staying home, you miss out on a lot of opportunities that could have made you happier. This can even make you feel worse and harbor more negative thoughts, which in turn, cause more negative feelings. You get stuck in a vicious cycle.

So, where do negative thoughts stem from? According to Dr. Aaron Beck, a psychiatrist at the University of Pennsylvania and pioneer of cognitive behavioral therapy, negative thinking patterns are rooted from childhood. Negative thoughts are fixed and automatic.

If a child does not get much affection from his parents, he might go to great lengths just to please them. His parents may praise him for his good work in school. This kind of thinking may help him for a certain period of time. However, as he grows older, he may experience things that are beyond his control and this may cause him to go back to his negative thinking patterns.

Through cognitive behavioral therapy, he may understand that his negative thinking patterns are not healthy and helpful for his growth. He may learn coping skills that he can use to overcome fears, panic, and anxiety. With continued treatment, he may eventually overcome his negative thoughts and become a more rational person.

While it is true that negative things happen, you should not allow them to take over your life. When you are in a disturbed state of mind, your interpretations and predictions can make it difficult for you to deal with your situation. Cognitive behavioral therapy encourages individuals to evaluate real-life experiences and test strategies to see if they can be beneficial to them. It also helps them correct their misinterpretations.

Types of Cognitive Behavioral Therapy

The British Association of Behavioral and Cognitive Psychotherapies state that behavioral and cognitive psychotherapies are based on principles and concepts that have been derived from psychological models of behavior and emotion. They include various treatment methods.

The following are the different types of therapeutic methods that make use of cognitive behavioral therapy:

Rational Emotive Behavior Therapy (REBT)

It focuses on identifying and changing irrational beliefs. It involves determining the underlying irrational belief, actively challenging such belief, and recognizing and changing irrational thoughts.

Cognitive Therapy

It focuses on identifying and changing distorted or inaccurate thinking patterns, behaviors, and emotional responses.

Dialectical Behavior Therapy

It deals with behaviors and thinking patterns that make use of strategies such as mindfulness and emotional regulation.

Multimodal Therapy

It states that psychological issues have to be treated by addressing the seven modalities, namely behavior, sensation, affect, imagery, drug or biological considerations, cognition, and interpersonal factors.

Components of Cognitive Behavioral Therapy

It is common for people to have feelings and thoughts that compound or reinforce faulty beliefs, which often cause problematic behaviors that affect the different aspects of life, such as personal relationships, career, academics, and health.

For example, an individual who has low self-esteem may harbor negative thoughts regarding his appearance or abilities. Because of this, he may avoid social situations and miss out on opportunities for career advancement.

Through cognitive behavioral therapy, he may combat destructive behaviors and thoughts. His therapist can help him identify problematic beliefs during the functional analysis stage. During this time, he learns how his feelings, reactions, and thoughts lead to maladaptive behaviors. This process can be difficult, particularly for individuals with introspection problems. Nevertheless, it can ultimately bring about insights and self-discovery that are vital for treatment.

Cognitive behavioral therapy also focuses on the specific behaviors that cause problems. In this stage, the patient learns and practices new skills that are useful in real-world scenarios. For example, an individual who suffers from drug addiction can practice new coping mechanisms and rehearse ways on how to deal with or avoid social situations that might trigger a relapse.

In a lot of cases, cognitive behavioral therapy is a gradual approach that helps people take the necessary steps towards behavioral change. For instance, a person who suffers from social anxiety may begin by visualizing himself in a situation that induces anxiety. Then, he may start to practice conversations with family and friends. As he progressively works towards his goal, he finds the process less daunting and his goals easier to attain.

CHAPTER 2

21 PRACTICAL WAYS TO DEAL WITH ANXIETY, DEPRESSION, WORRY, FEAR, AND PANIC

Everybody experiences anxiety, depression, worry, fear, and panic once in a while. Unexpected situations and events are normal occurrences in life. Whenever you experience an unpleasant sensation or feeling, you should do your best to overcome it.

First, you have to recognize what you are feeling. Then, you have to accept it and find a way to move on from it. Do not attempt to ignore or deny your anxiety, depression, worry, fear, or panic because this would just delay your recovery.

To help you out, here are some techniques you can use to improve your condition and make you feel better. These are simple and straightforward strategies that you can do on your own each time you have an episode.

1. Listen to upbeat music.

Music is said to be food for the soul. Listening to upbeat tunes can instantly change your atmosphere and create a positive vibe. It is also a great way to pass the time, relax, and entertain yourself. More importantly, it can help reduce your stress and anxiety as well as lower your blood pressure and boost your immune cell count.

A song with cheerful lyrics or music with an upbeat tone can effective alter your brain chemistry and boost your mood levels. In fact, researchers have found this theory to be correct. David Lewis-Hodgson, a researcher in the United Kingdom, has found that listening to the song Weightless by Marconi Union can reduce anxiety by 65%. How cool is that?

Other researchers also recommend listening to Celtic, Native American, and Indian stringed-instruments, drums, and flutes to alleviate stress and anxiety. According to researchers at

17

Stanford University, listening to music can alter brain function just like medication.

In addition, they have found that any form of music with sixty beats per minute may cause the brain synchronize with its beats and produce alpha brainwaves. Hence, upbeat music can improve the mood and induce optimism. Fast music can improve your concentration skills. Slow music can quiet your mind and relax your body muscles. In essence, listening to good music can significantly enhance your wellbeing.

2. Distract yourself.

Anxiety, worry, and panic often cause overthinking, which in turn, leads to more anxiety, worry, and panic. In order to remove yourself from this vicious cycle, you have to find a way to distract yourself from harmful and unhelpful thoughts.

The human mind is powerful. You become what you think. So, if you always have negative thoughts, you will grow up to be a pessimistic person. If you always have negative self-talk, your self-confidence and self-esteem levels will be low. Your thoughts can be your greatest enemy when depression starts to set in.

This is why you have to remind yourself that you are the master of your own thoughts. You can control what you think and how you feel about everything. If something happens and your anxiety is triggered, you should distract yourself to take your mind off this trigger.

For instance, you can go out for a walk, watch a TV show, or play with your pet. You can have a snack, complete a puzzle, or play a video game. Do anything that can take your mind off worries and fears. Staying busy is an effective way to stay away from harmful and unhelpful thoughts.

3. Connect with family and friends.

People who undergo depression often want to be left alone. They isolate themselves because they do not feel like talking to anyone. However, isolating yourself from others is not a good idea because it will only make your situation worse.

If you are going through difficult times, you have to reach out to other people. Call your friends or visit your family members. Interacting with your loved ones is good for your wellbeing.

Researchers have found that strong social bonds can strengthen mental health. As much as possible, you should opt for face-to-face interactions rather than merely phone calls and digital communication.

According to Dr. Alan Teo, researcher at VA Portland Health Care System and assistant professor of psychiatry at the Oregon Health and Science University, conversations via phone and the Internet are not as powerful as conversations in person when it comes to alleviating depression.

In the study he conducted with his colleagues, he has found that the participants who saw their friends and family at least three times a week were able to reduce their symptoms of depression by 6.5%.

4. Talk to a counselor, mentor, or anyone you trust.

Talk to a person you trust so that you can feel comfortable opening up. You may talk to a close friend who may relate to what you are going through or a family member who may give you support. You may also talk to a social worker who is trained to deal with issues like yours as well as a counselor. If you are religious, you may also speak with a priest, a rabbi, or anyone you look up to.

Ideally, the people you talk to should be outside your situation. This means that they should not be involved in whatever you are going through so that they may give you unbiased advice. They should also be neutral and not judgmental. Counselors are effective because they were trained to deal with various problems. Whatever you tell them will remain confidential, except for certain situations in which they are legally obliged or fear for safety.

Releasing your thoughts and feelings has a lot of benefits. For instance, it lets you sort through feelings. When you talk out loud about what is going on inside you, you clarify everything that worries you. Speaking out loud makes your fears less powerful. Sorting through your feelings allows you to know more about what you are dealing with. Keeping your thoughts and feelings to yourself only make you more confused.

Talking to another person also helps you release tension and put things in perspective. You may not realize it, but carrying worries, fears, and doubts creates physical tension. Getting them off your chest can do wonders for your health. Moreover, telling someone about what bothers you can make your problems less overwhelming. You can gain a fresh perspective from the other person, which can help you deal with your situation more objectively.

5. Recite positive affirmations.

Give yourself positive self-talk. The things you tell yourself become ingrained in your memory. So, you should tell yourself good things so that you can improve your thoughts, feelings, behaviors, and quality of life.

Depressed individuals tend to view the world negatively. They often blame themselves when things go wrong and they attribute good things to luck. They do not believe in themselves. Their depression reinforces feelings of worthlessness and self-doubt.

Observe your self-talk and remind yourself that you are functional, loved, and worthy of great things in life. Refrain from taking your thoughts seriously whenever you are feeling low. Take note that acknowledging your thoughts do not necessarily mean that you believe them.

Give yourself positive self-talk every morning to start your day right. Once you get out of bed, you should head to your bathroom or dresser mirror to see your reflection. Talk to it as you stare at the reflection of your own eyes. Say nice things. Tell yourself how good you are and why you are worthy of a good life. Complimenting yourself in the morning will make you feel better and more energized to start your day.

Then again, see to it that your positive affirmations follow the right structure. They should be in the present tense, not in the past tense. This way, your mind will not go back to your old negative habits.

They should also consist of words with positive connotations. Refrain from using the words "not", "hate", and other words with negative connotations. Take note that your subconscious mind cannot tell the difference between positive and negative sentences.

So, for example, instead of saying "I do not like being late", you can say "I am always punctual" or "I am always on time". Instead of saying "I hate arguing with my family and friends", you can say "I enjoy maintaining a close relationship with my family and friends".

6. Write down positive statements or write in a journal.

You can carry index cards with positive statements to cheer you up whenever you are weary. You can also keep a jar filled with folded papers that contain positive quotes to uplift your spirits.

Write down the qualities or traits that you like about yourself. You can also ask others, such as your friends and family, to write what they like about you. Keep these as reminders of your amazing qualities. Each time you are feeling low, you can look at what you and others have written and instantly be reminded of how great a person you are.

Writing can also be therapeutic. You can keep a journal. Write down your thoughts, feelings, opinions, ideas, etc. Only you can read the entries, so you should be completely honest and carefree about what you write. Get everything off your chest and clear your mind.

7. Take a nap.

Have you ever heard someone tell you to "sleep on it" when you have a problem that bothers you. This may sound counterproductive since you want to deal with the problem right away. Napping or sleeping may seem like an attempt to avoid the problem.

However, napping is actually beneficial. In fact, it can boost your productivity and mental alertness. Hence, you can find more effective ways to deal with your problem. Taking a power nap can refresh both your mind and body. It prepares you to deal with more tedious tasks throughout your day.

Sleep helps the body recover from stress. It also allows it to repair itself. Ashley Merryman and Po Bronson also said that sleep promotes happiness. If you lack sleep, your hippocampus gets negatively affected. Thus, you forget good memories and recall bad ones.

Similarly, a study published in the BPS Research Digest shows that sleep influences sensitivity to negative emotions. The researchers have found that the participants who did not take their afternoon nap became more sensitive towards negative emotions such as fear and anger. On the other hand, the participants who took a nap became more sensitive towards positive emotions such as happiness.

What's more, napping increases energy as well as improves learning and memory. It promotes memory retention, prevents burnout, and reverses information overload. It even improves creativity and enhances your senses. So, if you are going through a rough patch, taking a nap can help you relax and improve your mind. When you wake up, you will have a better perspective and you will be able to deal with your situation more effectively.

8. Practice mindfulness.

Mindfulness has long been proven to be effective for alleviating depression, anxiety, worry, and panic. For centuries, people have practiced mindfulness to relax their mind and body so that they can be more efficient at doing their tasks and solving their problems.

Mindfulness is pretty easy to practice. It can be done at any time and any place. Look for a place where you can sit down in silence. You can sit on the floor or in a chair, but refrain from lying down as this might cause you to fall asleep. When you are settled, close your eyes and focus on the present moment. Refrain from having unnecessary thoughts. If a thought crosses your mind, simply acknowledge its presence and then let go. Do not judge or hold onto it. Bring your mind back to the present moment. Stay this way for several minutes. When you are done meditating, open your eyes and get up.

9. Practice anchoring.

Anchoring is a neuro-linguistic programming technique that helps people alleviate depression and anxiety. It encourages them to get their minds out of its negative state. Through this technique, you can be in the "zone" and feel good about yourself. Rather than feel helpless, stupid, and unattractive, you will feel worthy, smart, and appealing. You will be able to recognize your good characteristics and overcome the challenges that you face.

As its name implies, anchoring is about staying still. It puts you in a positive state of mind. To do it, you have to close your eyes and remember the moments in your life wherein you felt confident. Remember as many details as you can. As you visualize these moments, remember the way you felt during these times. Since these are positive memories, you may have likely felt confident, peaceful, and triumphant.

Recalling positive feelings can instantly boost your mood levels. Bask in the wonderful feeling you have. Then, you should turn everything upside down. Notice the way your body feels against your clothes and the floor. Use your visual, auditory, and kinesthetic senses to feel things inside and out. Likewise, use your senses to observe your environment.

Next, you have to make the OK sign using your hand. Touch the tip of your index finger to the tip of your thumb as if you are saying "OK" with a hand gesture. You also have to say the word "power" intensely. Say it as powerfully as you can. When you are done with these steps, you can open your eyes slowly and bring your awareness back to reality. You can now go about your day with more confidence and energy.

10. Celebrate small wins.

Do not just focus on big wins; celebrate small wins as well. After all, little things lead to great things. Karl Weick, an author and former professor of Psychology, said that small wins are a series of concrete and complete results of moderate importance. They are micro-goals that are easily attained.

When you gain small wins, you realize that you are capable of achieving things, regardless of how big or small they are. This mere realization can empower and motivate you to continue reaching for your goals. Remember that incremental improvements can lead to groundbreaking achievements.

To do this technique, you have to identify a major goal you have. Break it down into smaller and more digestible parts. Make sure that you also set specific deadlines and timeframes for every part. Do not forget to set a reward for every milestone as well. Once you complete a milestone, give yourself a treat to encourage you to go on and do better.

11. Stay away from social media.

If you cannot stay away from social media permanently, at least deactivate or log out of your account for a few days or weeks. Going off the grid can do wonders for your mental health.

Studies have found that social networking sites, such as Facebook, Instagram, and Twitter, can be detrimental to mental health if users do not know how to control themselves. People often compare themselves to others on social media in terms of career, money, and relationship success.

Dr. Karen North, director of the digital social media program and professor of communication at the University of Southern California's Annenberg School for Communication and Journalism, talked about a study on the effects of social comparison to mental health.

The study entitled Seeing Everyone Else's Highlight Reels: How Facebook Usage Is Linked to Depressive Symptoms was seen in the Journal of Social & Clinical Psychology. According to it, people become more depressed after spending a lot of time on social media, particularly after seeing their friends' updates and comparing themselves to their peers.

So, if you want to be happier and healthier, you should be content with your life and stop comparing yourself to others. Staying away from social media can help you appreciate yourself better. Focus on having a fulfilling life offline instead of online.

12. Practice COAL

Everyone has a critical inner voice that tries to get to their heads once in a while. It is the voice that tells you that you are worthless, stupid, or ugly. It is the voice that discourages you from trying new things, taking risks, and getting out of your comfort zone. It is the one that hinders your progress. This negative voice is harmful and detrimental to success and happiness.

To challenge your critical inner voice, you have to see yourself for who you really are. Be more aware of your feelings, thoughts, goals, and values. Dr. Dan Siegel recommends practicing the COAL approach. It is about being Curious, Open, Accepting, and Loving towards yourself and experiences as opposed to being critical.

13. Meditate or pray.

If you are religious, you can turn to religion to increase your sense of self-worth. Praying to your deity can help you gain peace of mind. According to Dr. Jennifer Crocker, a researcher, turning to something that you consider to be bigger than yourself is effective in increasing your sense of self-worth and alleviating anxiety, stress, and depression.

However, if you are not religious, you can simply meditate. For a lot of people, meditation helps them improve their spirituality as well as strengthens their mind and body. There are different types of meditation you can choose from. Choose whatever feels right for you and stick with it if it helps you alleviate anxiety, depression, panic, and worry.

14. Practice self-hypnosis.

Hypnosis has been practiced for centuries to help people conquer their fears. It is an effective way to change your beliefs and make them more rational. It involves digging deep into the subconscious to get rid of damaging beliefs and habits that prevent success and growth. It also involves putting people into a trance to make them more susceptible to suggestions.

The principles of hypnosis and self-hypnosis are the same. With self-hypnosis, however, you get to work by yourself. There is no need for you to work with a hypnotherapist. Self-hypnosis actually lets you respond more easily and effectively to hypnotherapeutic suggestions as well as reinforce and consolidate the therapeutic benefits of hypnotherapy.

In order for self-hypnosis to be effective, you need to believe in it. Otherwise, you will contradict the process. You also have to stay in a place that is quiet, clean, comfortable, and free from distractions.

You can go to a quiet room and sit in a chair. You can also lie down on a couch. As you sit or lie down, you should turn your attention to a specific object. This can be anything, such as a pendulum or pen. Stare at it for a while. Then, you should close your eyes and take deep breaths.

Turn your focus to your breathing. With every breath you take, you should feel your body relax more. Think of the stress and tension in your body and visualize them dissipating from your muscles. Visualize them exiting your system. Next, you should recall the object of your focus. Visualize it moving back and forth. Allow this image in your head to relax your mind.

Start counting down from 10 to 1. As you count down, remind yourself that you are going deeper into the hypnosis process. Remember that once you reach 1, you will be in a trance. Then, once you are done with the process, you should start counting back up. Count from 1 to 10 and tell yourself to wake up refreshed and rejuvenated. Finally, open your eyes, wake up from the trance, and get on with your day.

15. Use the Superman pose.

The Superman pose is one of the most commonly used power poses. According to Amy Cuddy, associate professor and social psychologist from Harvard University, the use of high and low power poses can affect self-confidence levels. In her study, the participants who held high power poses during an interview did better than those who held low power poses.

In conclusion, people who hold high power poses, such as a superhero pose, take more risks, which affect their physiology. They also have lower cortisol levels and higher testosterone levels.

To do the Superman pose, you have to stand up straight and align your shoulders. Hold your head up high, place your hands on your waist, and keep your feet apart. Hold this pose for a couple of minutes or until you feel power flow throughout your body. Take deep breaths. Each time you feel anxious or nervous, do the Superman pose to give you a confidence boost.

16. Stand up straight.

Richard Petty from Ohio University and Pablo Brinol from the Universidad Automonma de Madrid conducted a study and found that people who sit up with their backs straight are more likely to be optimistic than those who do not.

So, if you are not feeling the Superman pose, you can simply stand up straighter. Good posture boosts confidence. Slouching, on the other hand, makes you seem unsure of yourself. You will feel more empowered when you keep your back straight and your chin up.

17. Occupy more space.

Olivia Fox Cabane, executive coach and author, recommends taking up a bigger space when you talk or interact with other people. Occupying more space can make you look more dominant and feel more empowered.

So, when you are in a party or social event, do not be afraid to spread out your arms or move around. When you are engaging in a conversation with someone, feel free to keep your feet apart and make hand gestures. Do not restrict yourself to a tiny space because this would just make you feel smaller and lower your self-confidence.

Likewise, when you are walking on the sidewalk, you should stay in the center instead of on the sides. This way, you can take up more space and increase your level of confidence.

18. Smile

Smiling can make you feel good as well as brighten other people's day. In fact, smiling becomes more effective when you think positive thoughts at the same time.

In a study done at Michigan State University, researchers have found that customer service department employees who fake their smiles end up having worse moods at the end of the day. They also become more withdrawn and less productive at work. On the other hand, employees who smile genuinely end up having higher mood levels and more productivity.

Moreover, smiling can help alleviate pain and reduce distress. Psychologists refer to this as the facial feedback hypothesis. You get to reap the benefits of smiling even if you only force it. So, you should try to smile even though you do not feel like doing it.

Then again, isn't this contradictory to the previous study? No, it is not. There is a difference between forcing yourself to smile to be happier and faking a smile while harboring negative thoughts. So, if you want to be happier and healthier, you should smile more often.

19. Practice gratitude.

Whenever you are feeling weary, just think of the things that you have and be grateful. Sometimes, all you need to do is recognize your blessings to boost your mood. Once you realize how much goodness you have, you will be happier.

Oftentimes, people neglect the good things that they have because they are used to seeing them all the time. They forget to be grateful for their family, friends, job, home, food, water, and even the air they breathe.

They forget to appreciate these good these because they are so focused on wanting to acquire more.

When you practice gratitude, you instantly uplift your spirits and reduce your risk of depression. In a study published in the Journal of Happiness, it was found that the participants who wrote letters of gratitude for three weeks increased their levels of happiness and decreased their symptoms of depression.

It is easy to practice gratitude. Simply think of the people that you are glad to have in your life. Look around you. Look at the things that keep you happy and satisfied. Do not ignore the little things because they also matter. Everything that you have is a blessing in your life; so, you should be grateful. Practice gratitude upon waking up in the morning and before going to bed in the evening.

20. Perform breathing exercises.

Every time you feel stressed, you should pause for a moment and take deep breaths. Abdominal breathing, also known as diaphragmatic breathing, involves inhaling and exhaling in a way that makes the diaphragm move up and down.

Researchers at Harvard Medical School said that you can feel anxious and unhappy when your tiny blood vessels get deprived of air. Deep breathing stimulates the parasympathetic system, which helps the body relax and alleviate stress.

When you are relaxed, your heart rate and blood pressure go down. Your digestion gets better and you sweat less. If you make taking deep breaths a habit, you train yourself to turn off your fight or flight response. This, in turn, causes you to be more present and clear with your thoughts.

Furthermore, you should remember that breathing is connected to emotions. In a study conducted by Pierre Phillipot, it was found that the different emotional states are connected to distinct respiration patterns. So, whenever you are stressed, anxious, angry, or feeling out of control, you should perform breathing exercises to calm yourself and feel better.

21. Exercise

Physical exercise has long been known to help improve the mind and body. Aside from toning muscles, it also helps boost mood levels and alleviate symptoms of anxiety and depression.

In a study published in the Journal of Sport and Exercise Psychology, it was found that endorphin-boosting and heart-pumping workouts can promote happiness.

According to researchers, people who are physically active experience more feelings of enthusiasm and excitement than those who are sedentary inactive. Dr. David Muzina, founding director of the Cleveland Clinic Center for Mood Disorders Treatment and Research, said that exercise stimulates the production of brain chemicals that fight against depression.

Running is one of the most recommended exercises for improving mood. According to a 2014 study, it can even lengthen your lifespan. Running causes long term changes in the norepinephrine and serotonin, which are the neurotransmitters responsible for your positive feelings. Its repetitive motions also have a meditative effect on your brain.

In a review published in the Journal of Psychiatry and Neuroscience, researchers discovered that exercise is just as effective as antidepressants when it comes to alleviating depression. Moreover, running can help you sleep better at night as well as lower your stress levels.

Aside from running, you can also try hiking. This is great because it lets you exercise your body and enjoy the wonders of nature at the same time. You can take a hike in the woods, for example.

Nature has a calming effect. Being around trees and plants can help reduce your anxiety and stress. A study published in Environmental Health and Preventive Medicine in 2009 has shown that people who take a walk in the woods for twenty minutes can lower their stress levels.

In a similar research, it was found that immersing in nature has positive effects on mental health. The participants who took a walk in nature for fifty minutes were able to improve their memory function and reduce their anxiety.

Then again, if you prefer to stay indoors, you can try yoga. In a study published in Evidence-Based Complementary and Alternative Medicine in 2007, it was found that the participants who practiced yoga were able to significantly reduce their depression, anxiety, anger, and neurotic symptoms.

In a similar study done in 2012, the researchers found that the participants who did yoga were able to reduce their symptoms of anxiety and stress.

Yoga is more than just strengthening the core and stretching. It is also about focusing on breathing. It slows down and calms the mind.

CHAPTER 3

HOW TO PREVENT
SMOKING

Smoking is dangerous for the health. In fact, it is not just dangerous for the smoker. Secondhand smoke is also dangerous for anyone who gets exposed to it. This is why smoking should be avoided.

There are plenty of ways on how to prevent smoking, such as by increasing the tax on tobacco products and having stricter laws on who can buy tobacco products as well as where, when, and how they can be bought. There can also be restrictions on advertisements and health warnings on cigarette packages.

Nonetheless, preventing should not only take place in the workplace, at schools, or in communities. It should also take place in your home and everywhere you go. You have to discipline yourself to avoid smoking by doing the following:

Strategies for Preventing Smoking

Create a quit plan.

Your day can flow more smoothly if you have a plan. Having a quit plan lets you stay confident, motivated, and focused on quitting. You can create your own quit plan or search for a readymade quit program online. You can also call a quitline to help you get started.

Also, you can check out various quit methods that may help you achieve your objectives. Take note that not every method works for everyone. What works for someone else may not exactly work for you. You have to use a quit plan that fits your specific needs and requirements.

Keep yourself busy.

Staying busy is a good way to prevent or quit smoking. It can help you take your mind off cigarettes or tobacco products. It can distract you from such unhealthy cravings.

There are a variety of ways on how you can keep yourself busy. For example, you can go for a walk in the park, exercise at your local gym, chew hard candy or gum, watch a movie, read a book, or immerse yourself in your work.

Change your routine.

If you often smoke after a meal, then you should change your routine. For instance, you can go straight to doing the dishes or sit down in a non-smoking area.

Ideally, you should identify the times when you start to crave for a smoke. Take note that a craving usually lasts for five minutes. So, you should think of strategies that last for five minutes, such as dancing, singing, or taking a walk. If you are at a party, you should leave before you get a chance to smoke.

Avoid smoking triggers.

If you are trying to recover from smoking, you should refrain from exposing yourself to possible triggers, such as things, places, situations, and people that may urge you to smoke. Avoiding these triggers is an effective way to prevent smoking.

To avoid triggers, you should throw away anything that is related to smoking, such as cigarettes, tobaccos, ash trays, matches, and lighters. Refrain from consuming caffeinated products because they can make you jittery. Drink more water.

Avoid going or passing by places that remind you of smoking such as stores that sell cigarettes and bars frequented by people who smoke. You should only go to restaurants and other places where smoking is not allowed. Likewise, you should avoid hanging out with smokers. Inform your family and friends about your decision to avoid smoking so that they won't smoke in your presence.

See to it that you live a healthy lifestyle. Eat nutritious foods and get sufficient amounts of rest and sleep. Exhaustion can cause you to start smoking. You should also modify your routine so that you can avoid anything that might lead you to smoking.

Be particular about your diet. According to a study, foods such as meats can make cigarettes taste more satisfying. This is why a lot of people tend to smoke after eating dinner. Conversely, there are foods that can make cigarettes taste terrible such as fruits, vegetables, and cheese. So, instead of eating burgers and steaks, you may want to eat veggie pizza.

Likewise, there are beverages that tend to make cigarettes taste better such as coffee, tea, soda, alcohol, and sparkling drinks. So, if you want to avoid smoking, you should opt for juice or water.

Look for replacements.

If you want to increase your chances of success, you should undergo nicotine replacement therapy. Here, you will be taught how to use patches, tablets, gums, nasal sprays, and lozenges to replace cigarettes and tobaccos. You can also use e-cigarettes and inhalators.

Another trick is to keep your smoking hand busy. If you usually use your right hand to smoke, you should hold something else using this hand. For example, you can carry a purse, a book, or a mineral water bottle. This way, you can refrain from reaching for a stick of cigarette.

You can also keep your mouth busy by drinking from a straw or munching on a snack. If your hands and mouth are busy doing something else, you can reduce your likelihood of smoking.

List down your reasons for wanting to prevent or quit smoking.

Why do you want to prevent or quit smoking? Everyone has a different reason for making changes. Your reasons might include your family, significant other, finances, or health.

Whatever your reasons are, you should think of them often. Remind yourself of these reasons by posting photos or sticky notes all over your home or office. For example, if your reason for wanting to prevent or quit smoking is your baby, you can keep a photo of her on your desk. Each time you get an urge to smoke, just take the photo and look at it so that you can be reminded of why you want to make such changes.

Get help and support.

Willpower alone may not be enough to prevent smoking. So, you may want to seek help from other people, such as your family and friends as well as mental health professionals.

Inform your family and friends about the changes that you are making in your life. Tell them that you need their help and support so that you can be completely smoke-free for the rest of your life. Tell them exactly what you need from them. Your loved ones can help you go through challenging times.

Of course, trained professionals can also support and assist you. Therapists, counselors, and social workers have the educational background, skills, and experiences that are necessary to help you prevent or quit smoking. You may also call the NHS Smokefree helpline.

Remain optimistic.

Quitting and preventing smoking is not easy. It cannot be done overnight. You need to have the patience and discipline to succeed. Expect to go through rough spots, especially in the first few days. You have to stay strong during these times. Remind yourself that you are worthy and capable of living a smoke-free life.

Stay positive throughout the process. Be generous to yourself as well. Treat yourself to rewards for your efforts at staying smoke-free. Refrain from beating yourself up when you have a relapse. Learn from your mistake and do your best to avoid giving in to the urge to smoke.

CHAPTER 4

HOW TO PREVENT
ADDICTIONS

Addiction ruins lives. It prevents people from forming and maintaining relationships, being productive at work and/or school, and functioning normally in society. So, before it becomes too late, you should find ways on how to prevent yourself from being addicted to illegal drugs, alcohol, and other things.

One way to prevent addiction is through intervention and screening. Prevention has to start in childhood and continue in adolescence. This way, addiction can be successfully prevented in adulthood.

Strategies for Preventing Addictions

There is a variety of strategies you can use to prevent addictions. These strategies should be employed in order to help old and young people understand the implications of using illegal substances and prevent them from making a negative impact in their lives.

In schools and communities, for example, addiction can be prevented by teaching children and adolescents to resist social pressure. They should be taught that they do not have to go along with their peers in order to belong. They can be independent and still make friends. They should also be taught how to improve their self-esteem, manage their anxiety and stress, and improve their communication and decision-making skills.

Taxes should also be increased for alcohol and tobacco products. In addition, the availability of excess prescription medications should be reduced. Advertisements and marketing of addictive substances should be restricted as well.

Self-Help Tips on How to Prevent Addictions

For the past years, researchers have tried to discover what causes people to develop addictions to substances or behaviors. They have found that all addictions trigger a neurological response that activates the reward system in the brain. This causes an addicted individual to crave more of his addiction.

Sadly, there are certain things that can never be changed when preventing addiction. These include family history, past trauma, and childhood environment. All of these factors contribute to the way a person thinks, feels, and behaves. They also contribute to their anxiety, depression, and addiction.

Fortunately, there are still plenty of ways on how you can deal with your anxiety, stress, or depression. Likewise, there are still lots of ways on how you can prevent addiction. Here are some of them:

Deal with past trauma and pain.

If your past is haunting or bothering you in the present, you have to face it and deal with it head on. Ignoring or repressing it will only make your condition worse. You need to deal with whatever is coming back from the past to mess with your present. Read self-help books and attend support groups. If necessary, you should work with a therapist to help you deal with past trauma and hurts.

Seek help from professionals.

If you are impulsive, lack self-control, are antisocial, or are aggressive, you should seek professional assistance. The National Institute on Drug Abuse recommends working with a therapist to help you deal with drug or alcohol abuse. You can also speak with a counselor regarding your intense sensations and extreme experiences.

Surround yourself with supportive people.

You can get better faster if you have adequate support from your loved ones, mental health professionals, and other people. This is especially true if you are part of the lesbian, gay, bisexual, transgender, or queer (LGBTQ) community. According to the Centers for Disease Control, the members of this community are more likely to use and abuse drugs or alcohol. They turn to these substances in an attempt to deal with their self-esteem issues, trauma, and other problems.

Choose your friends wisely.

Peer pressure is present at any age. Even adults can be pressured into doing something. So, if you want to prevent addictions, you should refrain from hanging out with people who have them. This way, you can avoid being exposed to addictive substances as well as being encouraged to use them.

Do not start young.

People who start using illegal substances or drinking at an early age are more likely to develop addictions later in life. If you have children or relatives who are teenagers, tell them to avoid using these substances and remind them of the consequences of using them. Spread the word about addiction to help more people avoid it.

Learn about the consequences of addiction.

You may not realize the consequences of your actions. Once you do, however, you may have a change of heart. Once you find out what happens to your mind and body as well as how your addiction can affect your loved ones, you may be motivated to change your ways.

Form strong connections.

Sometimes, all you need are people who care about you. You may just need a friend to talk to about your woes. Once you develop friendships, you may no longer feel the need to turn to drugs or alcohol to drown your sorrows. When you have people who support and listen to you, you can feel more at peace.

Take part in anti-drug, alcohol, and tobacco programs in your community.

According to researchers, these programs are effective in helping people change their ways and maintain their new lifestyles. These early intervention programs can help people prevent risky behaviors.

Determine your personal triggers.

Everyone's triggers are different. For some individuals, getting drunk or high is the direct result of anxiety or stress. For others, it is the result of hanging out with friends who like to drink at bars.

In order to determine your personal triggers, you have to ask yourself when you think about alcohol or drugs the most. Find out which situations make you more likely to use and abuse these substances. Identify what your reasons are for using them. Do you use them to momentarily forget about pain or responsibilities? Do you use them to release stress?

Once you get the answers to these questions, you should plan a way to work on them. You have to determine trigger situations when they occur so that you can take the necessary steps to stay away from them.

Avoid stress.

Stress is one of the most common reasons why people turn to alcohol, nicotine, and illegal drugs. They say that they just want to release stress.

So, if you want to prevent addictions, you should avoid getting stressed in the first place. To avoid it, you can practice breathing exercises. Close your eyes and take deep breaths. You can also distract yourself by engaging in enjoyable activities. You can also turn to exercise to release feel good chemicals in your body and feel better immediately.

CHAPTER 5

HOW TO OVERCOME
PHOBIAS

It is normal for people to have certain irrational fears. Some people are afraid of heights. Others are afraid of spiders. These fears are often minor for a lot of people. However, when your fears become so intense that they bring about anxiety, they might be phobias.

What Are Phobias?

Phobias are intense fears of certain things, people, or situations that do not really pose danger in reality. Some of the most common fears and phobias include heights, flying, needles, and closed-in places. Most phobias are developed in childhood, but there are also phobias that are developed in adulthood.

If you have phobias, you may already know that your fears are irrational. Nevertheless, you are still not able to control them. Simply thinking about your feared situation or object is enough to make you feel anxious. When you

74

get exposed to your fears, you experience overwhelming terror.

Most people go to great lengths just to avoid the object of their fears. This causes them to miss out on a lot of things or even put themselves at risk or in danger. If you want to live a more satisfying and stress-free life, you have to deal with your fears. Your first step is to acknowledge that you have fears and determine whether they are normal or irrational.

Normal Fears versus Irrational Fears

Phobias are irrational fears. Experiencing fear in dangerous situations is normal and may even be helpful. Your fears may protect you when they activate your fight or flight response. When your mind and body gets ready for action, you are able to respond quickly to threats. You are able to protect yourself.

However, threats are not really present with phobias. These irrational fears merely exaggerate the intensity or severity of the object of fear. For example, it is normal for people to be afraid of large dogs with large teeth. These dogs can really become vicious, after all. Then again, it is irrational to be afraid of puppies or poodles. These dogs are small and practically harmless. If you are still terrified of them, you may have a dog phobia.

So, how can you tell the difference between normal fears and irrational fears or phobias?

Your fear is normal when you feel anxious whenever you take off during storms or fly through turbulence. Your fear is irrational when you avoid going to places because you have to ride an airplane to get there.

Your fear is normal when you get butterflies in your stomach whenever you climb a tall ladder or look down from the rooftop of a tall building. Your fear is irrational when you turn down good job opportunities because you have to work on the 11th floor.

Your fear is normal when you get nervous each time you see a Rottweiler or pit bull. Your fear is irrational when you avoid going to the park because you may see dogs.

Your fear is normal when you feel a bit queasy whenever your blood is drawn. Your fear is irrational when you avoid getting any medical treatment that involves needles.

Common Signs and Symptoms of Phobias

The signs and symptoms of phobias can range from mild anxiety to full blown panic attacks.

The closer you get to the object of your fear, the more fearful you become. You become even more fearful when you realize that getting away from it is difficult.

Some of the physical symptoms of phobias are:

- Difficulty breathing

- Sweating

- Tingling sensations

- Cold or hot flashes

- Churning stomach

- Lightheadedness or dizziness

- Shaking or trembling

- Chest pain

- Racing heart

- Some of the emotional symptoms of phobias are:

- Knowing that you are overreacting and yet still feeling powerless

- Feeling like you are going to pass out or die

- Fear of going crazy or losing control

- Feeling detached

- Feeling an intense need to run away or escape

- Feeling an overwhelming panic or anxiety

When to Seek Treatment

Even though phobias are pretty common, they do not always lead to distress. For example, people who have a snake phobia may not always encounter a snake if they live in the city.

If your phobia does not really affect your daily life, then you do not have to worry too much about it. However, if avoiding triggers or the object of your fear causes you to be less productive, less functional, and more anxious, then you have to do something about it.

You have to seek treatment if your phobia is preventing you from engaging in enjoyable activities and causing severe distress or disabling fear, panic, and anxiety. You also have to seek treatment if it causes you to avoid certain places, people, and situation as well as if it interferes with your day-to-day routine. You should also see a mental health professional if your phobia has been around more six months or more already.

Self-Help Tips on How to Treat Phobias

A combination of therapy and self-help can be effective in treating phobias. The following are some of the ways you can do to deal with your phobias:

Face your faces, one at a time.

You may want your fears to vanish all at once. However, this is not possible. Just like everything else in life, overcoming your fears involves several steps. You have to go through the entire process in order to get the results that you want.

When it comes to facing your fears, you have to be direct. Do not go around it just to avoid it. If you really want to get over your fear, you have to address it head on. There are things you can do to lessen its power or impact on you, such as researching about it. The more you know about it, the less fearful it can be. Soon, you will realize that the object of your fear no longer frightens or overwhelms you.

Gradual exposure is ideal. This method is known as desensitization. You have to expose yourself to the object of your fear gradually. This way, you can learn how to ride out your fear and anxiety until they disappear. As you repeatedly expose yourself to the object of your fear, you get used to it and you realize that it is not a huge threat after all. If your anxiety becomes intense, you have to withdraw. However, the next time you expose yourself to your fear, you have to push yourself a little further. Continue pushing yourself until you are no longer afraid of it.

For example, if you have a fear of spiders, you can start by looking at pictures of spiders and reading about them. Research about the different types of spiders. Find out how they live. Then, expose yourself to spiders by looking at them from afar. Eventually, you can come closer until you get the courage to hold one in your hands. When you do this, you will realize that spiders are pretty harmless and your fear of them was irrational.

Create a list.

List down the situations, people, or things that frighten you. For example, if you are fearful of flying, you should write down everything that is related to it. You can include booking a ticket, packing a suitcase, going to the airport, seeing airplanes take off, going through security, boarding the airplane, and listening to the announcements of flight attendants.

Be as clear and detailed as possible. This way, you can tackle each and every one of these factors. It is important to go through every factor so that you can completely face and eradicate your fears.

Build a fear ladder.

Organize the items that you wrote in your list. Arrange them from the one that scares you the least to the one that scares you the most. The item that is least scary should make you a bit anxious but not frightened or intimidated. Evaluate every item on your list and determine how you feel and think about it.

Make sure that you also think about your end goal. What do you wish to achieve from this list? For example, you may want to be in a huge crowd without getting a panic attack. Identify all the steps that you have to take in order to reach your end goal.

Practice.

Begin with the first step and do not go higher until you feel comfortable in that stage. You have to stay in a situation long enough for the anxiety to subside. Once you get comfortable in this stage, you can move higher on your fear ladder.

Also, you have to practice this strategy more often. The more you do it, the faster your progress can be. Just make sure that you move at your own pace. Do not rush the process.

Learn how to calm yourself.

Whenever you feel anxious or afraid, you experience a wide range of physical and emotional symptoms. Your heart may race and your palms may sweat. These sensations may already be frightening on their own. So, your fears may intensify and your phobia may become more distressing.

You have to learn how to calm yourself quickly so that you can be more confident in your ability to get through uncomfortable sensations. For instance, you can perform breathing exercises. When you are anxious, you tend to take shallow breaths. You have to watch yourself and be aware of your breathing. Once you sense anxiety creeping in, you have to pause for a while and take deep breaths from your abdomen. This way, your physical sensations will be reversed and your anxiety level will go down.

Stand or sit comfortably. Keep your back straight and place a hand on your chest. Place your other hand on your stomach and inhale slowly through your nose. As you breathe in, you should count up to 4. Notice the way your hand on your stomach rises.

Hold your breath for 7 counts, then exhale through your mouth for eight counts. As you breathe out, your abdominal muscles should contract. Inhale once more and repeat the process until you feel more relaxed. Perform deep breathing exercises for five minutes two times per day. Do these exercises each time you experience anxiety or fear.

CHAPTER **6**

HOW TO CHANGE CORE BELIEFS

Your beliefs are the truths that you hold on to and use to guide your life by. They can either trap or set you free. Since your beliefs can be powerful, you can get trapped by limiting beliefs. Likewise, you can be freed by rational ones.

Your core beliefs are your strongest beliefs. Once you open your awareness, you can find out who you truly are and why you think, feel, and act the way you do. You can also have more energy that you can use to change your life.

The process of changing your core beliefs may seem like a daunting task. After all, these beliefs have been in your system for a really long time. However, there are actually a lot of strategies you can use to change them.

Tips On How To Change Core Beliefs

See to it that you have the right core beliefs.

There are instances in which the core beliefs you think are causing the problem are not the really the ones that causes it. For example, you may think that you are an optimistic person. However, the truth is that you are actually quite pessimistic.

One way to determine if your core belief is right is by observing the way you talk to yourself in times of stress. If you catch yourself saying negative things, then you may be a negative person and this is the core belief that you have to change.

Identify your pattern. Evaluate your life up to this point. Did all your previous relationships fail? Did you always have arguments with your family and friends? Are you buried in debt? Once you identify your pattern, you should ask yourself what you think about it. Listen to your reasons. Then, ask yourself what you want and what you have to belief in order to get your desired results.

Have awareness.

The next step to changing your core beliefs is to have awareness. Observe the way you feel and act towards your beliefs. You will find it easier to change your old patterns when you see the way they affect your thoughts, reactions, and behaviors.

Simply understanding why you act the way you do may be enough to change your old patterns. However, if this is not enough for you, you may have to decide to "cancel" your thoughts. You should cancel thoughts that no longer serve your purpose. Cancel thoughts that you no longer find to be true.

Think about these thoughts and then release them. Then, think about your new beliefs. You have to be aware of your old thoughts so that you can effectively replace them with new ones. You also have to be aware of the triggers of your old thoughts. Keep in mind that these old beliefs were meant to protect you. Since you no longer need them, you have to let go of them.

Use a mirror.

Core beliefs such as "I do not deserve good things" and "I am unlovable" can be re-programmed by using a mirror. Get a mirror and look at your reflection. Tell yourself that you are lovable and that you deserve good things. Smile at your reflection. Look yourself in the eye.

Practice this technique daily until you become more confident about yourself and your abilities. As you repeatedly say positive statements to yourself, you rewire your subconscious mind.

You can also practice the mirror affirmation that Emile Coue developed in the 1900's. Stare at yourself in the mirror three times per day and recite the following three times:

"Every day, and in every way, I am getting better and better".

Saying this to yourself reprograms your subconscious and causes it to believe that your life does get better and better.

Learn from other people.

Research about the people you look up to and find out how they are able to change their core beliefs. Surely, they have talked about their processes in interviews. You can watch their videos or read articles about them so that you can find out how they think, what they tell themselves, and what they believe.

Use their process as guidelines for your own. Make them your inspiration to get better. If you are dedicated and disciplined, you will surely improve yourself as well.

Do not give up.

Do not give up until you get new core beliefs. At first, you may experience difficulties in changing your core beliefs. You may not be able to believe your new thoughts. The critical voice inside of you may contradict the positive statements you tell yourself.

When this happens, you have to stay strong. Remind yourself of your good qualities. Recall the instances in your life when you felt happy, loved, and successful. Knowing that you were able to have good things in the past can serve as a reminder that you can have more good things in the present and future.

Popular coach Tony Robbins said that personal breakthroughs start with a change of belief. You can effectively change your beliefs by making your brain associate pain with your old beliefs. You have to feel that these old beliefs brought about pain and sufferings in the past and that they are also affecting your present. Since you do not want to experience the same pain and sufferings in the future, you have to let go of these beliefs. You have to adopt new empowering beliefs that you can associate with pleasure and happiness.

CHAPTER 7

GOAL SETTING AND
MINDFULNESS

The power of intention is ideal to be used alongside goal setting. Blogger Dagmar Shoenrock recommends using the power of intention to increase your chances of achieving success. Your intent is the way you feel about your goals. When you set goals that you really want, you become more motivated to achieve them.

How To Connect Goal Setting With Mindfulness

The following steps can help you effectively connect goal setting with mindfulness:

Find your presence.

First of all, you need to find your presence. You have to stay true to yourself and stay present, regardless of the chaos around you.

When you hold a sense of presence, you stay in touch with your truest self or your essence.

Take deep breaths to stay focused in the present moment. Inhale slowly for five counts. Once you reach 5, you should pause for a while. Then, you should exhale slowly through your mouth for five counts. Repeat this process five times.

Calm your mind.

After performing breathing exercises, you can start to calm down your mind. Sit still and relax yourself. One session can last for ten minutes.

Get a timer and set it for ten minutes. Close your eyes. Stay comfortably in your position. Choose a feeling or word that you want to embody. For example, you can choose "peace", "success", "love", or "happiness".

Choose another word that you want to let go of. For example, you can choose "negativity", "fear", "anger", or "insecurity". When you inhale, you should silently recite the word that you want to embody. When you exhale, you should silently recite the word that you want to let go of. Repeat this process. Use these words as your mantra during your meditation session.

Connect with the heart.

Put one hand on your chest and think of your desires. Let your heart and mind come together. Allow them to help you achieve your dreams and desires. Observe the feelings, sensations, and emotions that they bring about.

Find out if certain dreams and desires come with joy, anxiety, excitement, or tension. If they either hold more negative or positive energy than others, you should stay with them for a while and notice whatever surfaces without judgment.

Mentally note the dreams and desires that you bring your excitement, motivation, and delight. Likewise, you should determine the ones that make you feel tense, fearful, or anxious.

Practice visualization.

Visualize yourself already having what you want. Select three dreams or goals that are associated with positive emotions.

Then, visualize them one by one. Be as vivid as possible. Imagine yourself achieving your goal and being happy with your success. Take note of every detail. How do you behave? How do other people react?

Spend a few minutes for every dream or goal visualization. Observe the way you feel as you visualize your future.

Practice affirmation.

Finally, you have to affirm your dreams or goals. Write them down. Feel positively about them. Include the positive emotions that you associate with your desires. Write down every detail, feeling, and motivation. Feel and believe that you will actually get what you want.

CONCLUSION

I'd like to thank you and congratulate you for transiting my lines from start to finish.

I hope this book was able to help you to learn about anxiety, depression, worry, and panic and the ways on how to deal with them. I hope that it was also able to give you sufficient information on cognitive behavioral therapy, how it works, and how it can help you deal with detrimental mental health issues and negative thoughts.

More importantly, I hope that I was able to cover all the fundamentals as well as encourage you to make positive changes into your life so that you can be happier, healthier, and more successful.

Remember that you can always improve yourself. If you want to have a healthier mind and body, make sure that you fight against stress, anxiety, and depression. Overcome your worries and fears.

Through this book, I hope that you found answers to your questions as well as learned more vital information. Mental health issues are no joke. They can truly be debilitating once they take over your life. Proper treatment is necessary. Nonetheless, there are also a lot of self-help techniques you can use aside from therapy.

Furthermore, you should take note that prevention is better than cure. So, before it gets too late, you have to prevent smoking and addictions. You also have to recognize your triggers so that you can also prevent anxiety, depression, worry, and panic.

The next step is to apply what you have learned from this book into your life. When you have a sound mind and body, you can live your life to the fullest.

I wish you the best of luck!

BONUS CONTENT

MENTAL TOUGHNESS

CHAPTER 1

Plato in his "Republic" talks about mental discipline. The Romans believed that men had to study certain subjects in order to become trained in the best traits of life which included basic intelligence, the right attitude towards things as well as core values. The subjects the Romans believed could bring about this type of mental fortitude were music, geometry, grammar, logic, astronomy, rhetoric and arithmetic. In Greco-Roman times these subjects were studied by rote and imitation. This lasted until quite recently and it was only later when pedagogues decided that this type of education was counter-productive and what was required was a "softer" type of education based on moral values and the humanities studies were brought to the fore, however, we will not deal with this and will deal with the basics about mental discipline which in our times is seeing a resurgence in modern thinking.

Today mathematics is seen to be a mental discipline and the idea is to transpose mathematical thinking to common life thinking and problem solving.

One of the ways to achieve mental discipline is to use mindfulness. This is a type of thinking that means we focus on what we are doing right now down to the finest detail. For example; eating. In mindfulness we would focus first on the table. Look at the table, see what its colours are, if it is wood, glass, iron or plastic. How high the table is. What it measures. What is on the table. The cutlery we are going to use to eat, the dishes, the different sets of dishes and cutlery for the other people that will be eating with us. Then we focus on the food. What exactly are we going to be eating. How we will be eating and we focus on our body, our arm reaching for the fork, the hand that grasps the fork, the fingers that hold it, the hand that goes down reaching for the food, the morsel that is placed on the fork. How the fingers, hand, arm and body move as we place the fork in our mouth with the food. The food. Is it hot or cold? Is it crunchy or soft? Does it drip. Is it salty or sweet? The colour of it. The odour of it. We chew it carefully extracting all the nutrition in it. We swallow. We focus all the time on the act of eating and we eat carefully, being and fusing ourselves with the act of nutrition. We are not distracted by other people, tv, a book, the radio, etc. We focus on the act of eating single minded. This is mindfulness and it can be applied to everything we do. By practicing mindfulness every day, we can reinforce our willpower and according to scientists, this can actually increase gravy matter in the brain.

Willpower is strengthened by mindfulness. Willpower is about the refusal to give in, to cave. Willpower is mindfulness in action. By meditating you create a calm space in your mind where your mind is not leaping from one thing to the next and with willpower you force your mind to stay still in the present. This is not easy. You must have tried meditating from time to time and all it did was two things: you got restless and left the meditation room or else you fell asleep. The way to meditate is to use mindfulness to calm your mind and anchor it to the present. Try to sit still and pay attention to what is happening around you or in you at this precise moment. Don´t get distracted. Just sit there and focus on what is happening right now. It is hard. Mental discipline is about doing this every single time you lose focus and this is where willpower comes in. Willpower is what will get you where you want to be every time your attention wanes. The best thing about willpower is that it can be fortified just like your mind because it is like a muscle and you can make it stronger.

Willpower is part of self-discipline. It is the essence of self-discipline. Forcing yourself to do things cannot be done without willpower. Willpower is the grease that the self-discipline machine uses to carry out the motions leading you to a better place inside yourself.

Willpower is what you need to strengthen in order to have mental discipline, it is one of the ingredients you need on your way to a more disciplined mind.

So, we have some things to use now right at the very beginning: mindfulness which is a form of willpower in baby steps. Willpower and these are attitudinal things that we need to use in our quest for mental discipline.

How do we get mental discipline?

There is no easy way to obtain mental discipline. It takes a lifetime to cultivate the mind. It is almost an art (remember the music, one of the subjects of the Romans that Plato talked about?). There is no way to buy yourself mental discipline. The only way is hard work so prepare for that. Make yourself a plan, a scheme, a way to tackle the issue. Use a notebook to write down all the things you will be doing and keep a sort of mental discipline diary. Read it every day.

Maybe you had a falling out in life, maybe something derailed you from your set path you had. Now while you are in your low moment, or contemplative moment, is the time to set the groundwork for your future which starts now (remember, mindfulness). Now is the time to ditch the old you that wasn't working and get yourself a new you (remember, attitudes). Make yourself abide by a new set of rules. There are ways in which you can use your daily living activities to have more self-discipline. One is getting up early. This doesn't seem like much but if you include it in your new you, it will make you start the day at a different hour and this in itself is going to have an impact on your day. Try it, if you get up at 8 in the morning, try getting up at 7 and see what the world looks like at that time of day. At first you will need almost all your willpower because when you open your eyes and see that it is still very early, your body will be begging you to snuggle down and stay in bed. Don´t. Get up and take a shower. Get yourself a coffee and once you have overcome the temptation to stay in bed and are actually in the kitchen preparing a coffee or a juice, give yourself a pat on the back. It will get easier as your mind adapts to your new schedule and, now that you have gotten up, what about using this extra hour for something special? Try meditation. Go into your living room or your porch with your coffee. If it is summer, sit out there in mindfulness taking in the sensations of the early morning. Stay out there for an hour, it won´t be wasted. Remember, you are rewarding yourself for having gotten up early and you got up early because you are on your way to having greater mental discipline. You are mapping out the steps you need to achieve your long-term goal and don´t forget to keep the forest in mind while focusing on the trees. This is a sample of what a person can do in an easy way to change his or her life.

Mental discipline is something you can learn but it is necessary to practice and repeat it a lot. This is the downside but if you use mindfulness as a tool, you can practice and repeat endlessly and effortlessly after a while because with mindfulness every time you do it is like the first time and this comes with an added thing, a Zen like quality that makes repetition pleasurable. If you practice a sport you will know what this is: it is hitting the ball perfectly every time like in tennis or the runner´s "high", the surge of dopamine in the brain helping you overcome the grind of repetition. If you make it a habit to observe yourself in a detached way while you are doing your practicing and repetition, you will develop your mindfulness and your self-discipline. There are ways that can help you achieve your self-discipline. One thing is to make it easy on yourself, eliminate things that suck your energy, that detract from your goal, for example, if you were dieting, eliminate the snacks and junk food. This is just common sense. It is not a good idea to go to the supermarket at lunch time. Use your common sense and eliminate the temptations that are going to undermine your self-discipline. If you get up in the morning early, do it. Get up and get away from the bed. Move. Go to the kitchen. Do something so you don´t crawl back into bed.

While considering snacks and junk food, remember to focus on healthy eating. This is part of the Spartan like training you will need to foster your mental-discipline so take it to another level and include proper eating in your routine.

Another element in getting mental discipline is to give yourself prizes for achieving things. Don´t make your quest for mental discipline a Marine training site because you will make things so difficult, so almost impossible to achieve that you will fail. Set yourself easy to achieve goals, gradually make them a little harder and set yourself up to win. This is a difficult thing. Lots of people who have decided to embark on achieving mental discipline to immure them from failure and disappointment do so because they have suffered a lot from failure and disappointment. One of the things to watch out for is the paradoxical thing which is: I fasted for one day and didn't eat anything. I am great. Then, immediately after, I rush out to McDonalds and have a binge… Why is this? This is because my mental discipline is so green and raw that I cannot withstand success and need to fail. Then we feel miserable and get all despondent and start considering Spartan discipline… this is wrong. The thing to do is to take it in stride.

Make room for failure and remember to immediately get up and start again or rather, continue. This is the key word: continue. The first time you have a major fail, you will throw this book out the window and go to bed feeling miserable because you failed. But if you go out and find this book and dust it off and read it again, the next time you fail will not be as bad. And this is the wonderful thing. Failing starts fading. Winning starts pushing failing to a side and one day during your mindfulness you will notice how you have changed.

Change: This is the secret to staying young forever. Change. The way in which you no longer do the things you used to do and now do new things or different ones. These are things to consider. If you let yourself change. If you are flexible and use your failings to change yourself, you will find ways in which your mental discipline will start having an effect on what you do every day. Experience is mindfulness in action. Mindfulness is mental discipline in action.

When you fail, which you will do, be sure to take note. Be disappointed, frustrated and angry but don´t forget the forest while you bash your head against the tree. Keep the forest in mind and go back. Get up early and dedicate some early morning silence to mindfulness and pick up where you left off.

118

Practice makes perfect and remember, the Greco-Romans prided themselves on rote learning. So you should too.